Keto Vegetarian Diet for a Healthy Lifestyle

Low-Carb Vegetarian Diet to Quickly Lose Weight and be Fit

Ricardo Abagnale

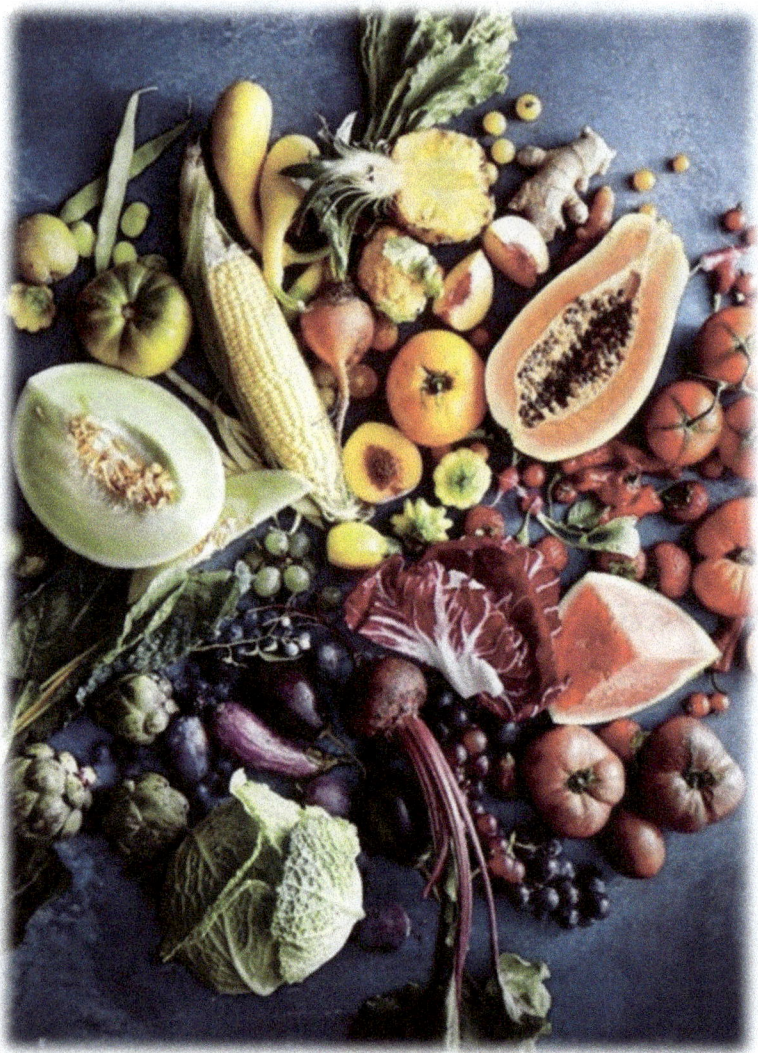

Table of Contents

INTRODUCTION 7

BREAKFAST **8**

PARSLEY SPREAD 8

BAKED CHEESY ARTICHOKES.. 10

MAINS **12**

ROASTED CAULIFLOWER AND BROCCOLI 12

CHEESY GRITS 14

CREAMY SQUASH SOUP.. 16

KETO CAESAR SALAD 18

CREAMY CUCUMBER EGG SALAD 20

ROASTED BROCCOLI WITH ALMONDS............................22

AVOCADO CILANTRO TOMATO SALAD 24

MEXICAN VEGAN MINCE 26

SIDES **28**

SAGE QUINOA..28

BEANS, CARROTS AND SPINACH SIDE DISH....................30

SCALLOPED POTATOES..33

SWEET POTATOES SIDE DISH....................................... 35

CAULIFLOWER AND BROCCOLI SIDE DISH...................... 37

WILD RICE MIX..39

RUSTIC MASHED POTATOES 41

FRUIT AND VEGETABLES **43**

FRESH FRUIT SMOOTHIE 43

POPOVERS 45

BROCCOLI, GARLIC, AND RIGATONI 47

VEGAN RICE PUDDING..49

CINNAMON-SCENTED QUINOA.. 51

SOUPS AND STEWS..**53**

PUMPKIN-PEAR SOUP 53

SWEET POTATO AND PEANUT SOUP WITH BABY SPINACH..............................56

TUSCAN WHITE BEAN SOUP..58

KETO PASTA...**61**

THAI TOFU SHIRATAKI STIR-FRY 61

CLASSIC TEMPEH LASAGNA..65

SALADS..**68**

YELLOW MUNG BEAN SALAD WITH BROCCOLI AND MANGO......................... 68

ASIAN SLAW 70

THE GREAT GREEN SALAD...72

SNACKS **74**

BAKED HOT SPICY CASHEWS SNACK 74

EASY AVOCADO AND CREMINI MUSHROOM MELTS 76

KETO HOT PEPPERS C.S...78

SPANISH VEGETABLE OMELET 80

ABSOLUTE AVOCADO PIZZA..82

ALMOND LEMON BISCUITS 84

DESSERTS **86**

LOW-CARB CURD SOUFFLÉ.. 86

CREAM CHEESE COOKIES... 88

CHIA SEEDS PUDDING WITH BERRIES 90

SMOOTHIE BOWL... 91

COCONUT MILK SMOOTHIE...92

YOGURT SMOOTHIE WITH CINNAMON AND MANGO 93

LEMON CURD DESSERT (SUGAR FREE) 94

CHOCOLATE ALMOND BUTTER SMOOTHIE...95

OTHER RECIPES..**96**

VEGAN GUMBO...96

EGGPLANT SALAD..98

CORN AND CABBAGE SOUP..100

OKRA SOUP 103

CARROT SOUP...105

BABY CARROTS AND COCONUT SOUP 107

INTRODUCTION

The Ketogenic diet is truly life changing. The diet improves your overall health and helps you lose the extra weight in a matter of days. The diet will show its multiple benefits even from the beginning and it will become your new lifestyle really soon.

As soon as you embrace the Ketogenic diet, you will start to live a completely new life.

On the other hand, the vegetarian diet is such a healthy dietary option you can choose when trying to live healthy and also lose some weight.

The collection we bring to you today is actually a combination between the Ketogenic and vegetarian diets. You get to discover some amazing Ketogenic vegetarian dishes you can prepare in the comfort of your own home. All the dishes you found here follow both the Ketogenic and the vegetarian rules, they all taste delicious and rich and they are all easy to make.

We can assure you that such a combo is hard to find. So, start a keto diet with a vegetarian "touch" today. It will be both useful and fun!

So, what are you still waiting for? Get started with the Ketogenic diet and learn how to prepare the best and most flavored Ketogenic vegetarian dishes. Enjoy them all!

Parsley Spread

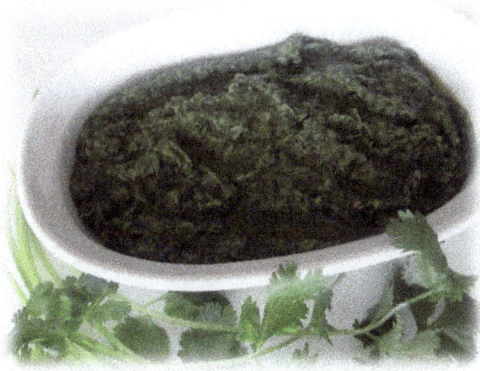

Preparation time: 5 minutes

Cooking time: 0 minutes

Servings: 8

Nutritional Values (Per Serving):

- calories 78
- fat 7.2
- fiber 1
- carbs 3.6
- protein 1.1

Ingredients:

- 1 cup parsley leaves
- 1 cup coconut cream
- 1 tablespoon sun-dried tomatoes, chopped
- 2 tablespoons lime juice
- ¼ cup shallots, chopped
- 1 teaspoon oregano, dried
- A pinch of salt and black pepper

Directions:

1. 1. In a blender, combine the parsley with the cream, the tomatoes and the other ingredients, pulse well, divide into bowls and serve for breakfast.

Baked Cheesy Artichokes

Preparation time: 10 minutes

Cooking time: 45 minutes

Servings: 6

Nutritional Values (Per Serving):

- calories 149
- fat 12.2
- fiber 4.3
- carbs 9.7
- protein 3.5

Ingredients:

- 1 cup spinach, chopped
- 1 cup almond milk
- 12 ounces canned artichokes, halved
- 2 garlic cloves, minced
- ½ cup cashew cheese, shredded
- 1 tablespoon dill, chopped
- A pinch of salt and black pepper
- teaspoons olive oil

Directions:

1. Heat up a pan with the oil over medium heat, add the garlic, artichokes, salt and pepper, stir and cook for 5 minutes.

2. Transfer this to a baking dish, add the spinach, almond milk and the other ingredients, toss a bit, bake at 380 degrees F for 40 minutes, divide between plates and serve for breakfast.

MAINS

Roasted Cauliflower and Broccoli

Preparation time: 10 minutes

Cooking time: 15 minutes

Servings: 12

Nutritional Values (Per Serving):

- Calories: 81
- Carbohydrates: 3.1 g
- Fat: 6.7 g
- Sugar: 1.1 g
- Cholesterol: 5 mg
- Protein: 1.9 g

Ingredients:

- 4 cups broccoli, florets
- 4 cups cauliflower, florets
- 6 cloves garlic, minced
- 2/3 cup Parmesan cheese, grated, divided
- 1/3 cup extra-virgin olive oil
- Pepper and salt to taste

Directions:

1. Preheat your oven to 450° fahrenheit. Spray with cooking spray a baking dish, then set it aside.
2. Add broccoli, cauliflower, half of the cheese, garlic, and olive oil into a mixing bowl and toss well to blend. Season with salt and pepper.
3. Arrange cauliflower and broccoli mixture in your prepared baking dish. Bake for 15 minutes in preheated oven.
4. Just before serving add remaining cheese on top. Serve hot and enjoy!

Cheesy Grits

Preparation time: 5 minutes

Cooking time: 8 minutes

Servings: 4

Nutritional Values (Per Serving):

- Calories: 388
- Cholesterol: 403 mg
- Sugar: 0.9 g
- Fat: 36.5 g
- Carbohydrates: 1.4 g
- Protein: 14.8 g

Ingredients:

- ½ cup butter, unsalted
- ½ cup vegetable broth
- ½ cup cheddar cheese, shredded

- 8 eggs, organic
- 1 teaspoon sea salt

Directions:

1. In a mixing bowl add your eggs, broth, and sea salt, mix well.
2. Melt butter in a pan over medium heat. Place your egg mixture into the pan and cook for 8 minutes or until the mixture thickens and curds form. Add the cheese to the pan and stir well.
3. Remove the pan from heat. Serve warm and enjoy!

Creamy Squash Soup

Preparation time: 10 minutes

Cooking time: 35 minutes

Servings: 8

Nutritional Values (Per Serving):

- Calories: 147
- Fat: 12.3 g
- Cholesterol: 10 mg
- Sugar: 1.6 g
- Carbohydrates: 7.7 g
- Protein: 3.2 g

Ingredients:

- 5 tablespoons extra-virgin olive oil
- 1 lb. butternut squash, peeled, diced
- 4 cups vegetable broth
- 3 garlic cloves, minced

- 2 bay leaves
- ½ cup heavy cream
- 1 teaspoon salt

Directions:

1. Heat 1 tablespoon of olive oil in a saucepan over medium heat. Add butternut squash, garlic, salt and sauté until lightly browned. About five minutes.
2. Add the broth, bay leaves and 4 tablespoons of olive oil into a saucepan. Bring to a boil. Simmer the squash for 30 minutes or until it is completely cooked. Discard the bay leaves.
3. Using blender puree the soup until smooth. Add heavy cream and stir well.
4. Serve warm and enjoy!

Keto Caesar Salad

Preparation time: 15 minutes

Servings: 8

Nutritional Values (Per Serving):

- Calories: 102
- Fat: 9.3 g
- Sugar: 0.8 g
- Cholesterol: 5 mg
- Carbohydrates: 2.3 g
- Protein: 3.3 g

Ingredients:

- 8 cups romaine lettuce, chopped
- 2 tablespoons lemon juice, fresh
- ¼ cup Parmesan cheese, grated, fresh
- ¼ teaspoon garlic powder
- 1 tablespoon mayonnaise

- ¼ cup extra-virgin olive oil
- ¼ teaspoon pepper

Directions:

1. In mixing bowl, combine olive oil, garlic powder, lemon juice and mayonnaise.
2. Add lettuce and cheese to the bowl. Season with pepper. Cover bowl and place in the fridge for about an hour.
3. Just before serving toss salad and enjoy!

Creamy Cucumber Egg Salad

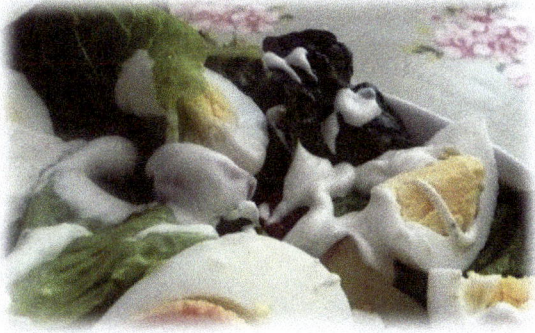

Preparation time: 15 minutes

Servings: 4

Nutritional Values (Per Serving):

- Calories: 176
- Fat: 12.7 g
- Cholesterol: 249 mg
- Sugar: 2.7 g
- Carbohydrates: 7.6 g
- Protein: 9.2 g

Ingredients:

- 6 eggs, organic, hard-boiled
- 1 medium cucumber, peeled, chopped
- 1 avocado, peeled, cubed
- ¼ cup mayonnaise
- ½ teaspoon paprika

Directions:

1. Peel and dice eggs.
2. In a bowl, mix ingredients well.
3. Serve and enjoy!

Roasted Broccoli with Almonds

Preparation time: 12 minutes

Cooking time: 20 minutes

Servings: 4

Nutritional Values (Per Serving):

- Calories: 206
- Fat: 15.7 g
- Sugar: 3.2 g
- Carbohydrates: 13 g
- Cholesterol: 7 mg
- Protein: 7.6 g

Ingredients:

- 1 ½ lbs. broccoli, cut into florets
- 1 tablespoon lemon juice
- 3 tablespoons olive oil
- 2 garlic cloves, sliced

- 3 tablespoons almonds, slivered, toasted
- ¼ teaspoon pepper
- ¼ teaspoon sea salt
- ¼ cup cheese, grated

Directions:

1. Preheat your oven to 425°Fahrenheit. Spray baking dish with cooking spray.
2. Add broccoli, garlic, oil, pepper, and salt in a mixing bowl and toss well.
3. Spread the broccoli in the prepared baking dish and roast in preheated oven for 20 minutes.
4. Add lemon juice, grated cheese, almonds over broccoli, toss well.
5. Serve hot and enjoy!

Avocado Cilantro Tomato Salad

Preparation time: 15 minutes

Servings: 4

Nutritional Values (Per Serving):

- Calories: 270
- Fat: 23.5 g
- Cholesterol: 0 mg
- Sugar: 5.4 g
- Carbohydrates: 16.6 g
- Protein: 3.6 g

Ingredients:

- 4 cups cherry tomatoes, halved
- 2 avocados, diced
- Juice of 1 lime, fresh
- ¼ cup cilantro, fresh, chopped

- 1 tablespoon extra-virgin olive oil
- Pepper and salt to taste

Directions:

1. In a mixing bowl add tomatoes, avocado, and cilantro.
2. In a small bowl, combine lime juice, olive oil, pepper, and salt.
3. Pour lime juice mixture over salad and mix well. Enjoy!

Mexican Vegan Mince

Preparation time: 5 minutes

Cooking time: 5 minutes

Serves: 4

Nutritional Values (Per Serving):

- Kcal: 232
- Fat: 16 g.
- Protein: 17 g.
- Carbs: 9 g.

Ingredients:

- 400 g Seitan Mince
- 2 cloves Garlic, minced
- 2 pieces Green Chili, chopped
- 2 tbsp Nutritional Yeast
- 1 tbsp Garam Masala
- 1 tsp Cumin Powder

- ½ tsp Salt
- 1 small Red Onion, diced
- 2 Roma Tomatoes, diced
- Cilantro for garnish
- 2 tbsp Olive Oil

Directions:

1. Heat olive oil in a non-stick pan. Add onions, garlic, and green chili. Sautee until aromatic.
2. Add mince and stir-fry for 3-5 minutes.
3. Add nutritional yeast, garam masala, and cumin powder. Stir until well combined.
4. Season with salt to taste.
5. Garnish with fresh cilantro and serve.

Sage Quinoa

Preparation time: 10 minutes

Cooking time: 30 minutes

Servings: 4

Nutritional Values (Per Serving):

- Calories 182
- Fat 1
- Fiber 1
- Carbs 11
- Protein 8

Ingredients:

- 1 tablespoon olive oil
- 1 yellow onion, chopped
- 1 cup quinoa

- 2 cups chicken stock
- 1 tablespoon sage, chopped
- 2 garlic cloves, minced
- A pinch of salt and black pepper
- 1 tablespoon chives, chopped

Directions:

1. Heat up a pan with the oil over medium-high heat, add the onion and the garlic and sauté for 5 minutes.
2. Add the quinoa and the other ingredients, toss, cook over medium heat for 25 minutes more, divide between plates and serve.

Beans, Carrots and Spinach Side Dish

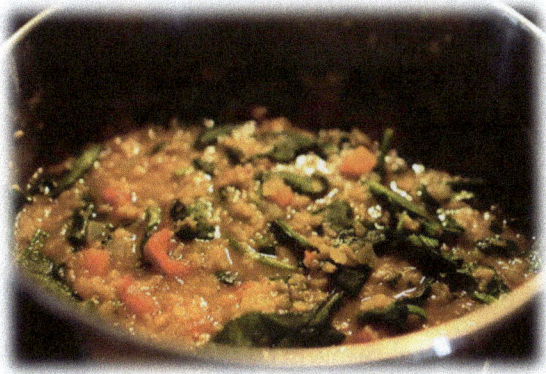

Preparation time: 10 minutes

Cooking time: 4 hours

Servings: 6

Nutritional Values (Per Serving):

- Calories 319
- Fat 8
- Fiber 14

- Carbs 43
- Protein 17

Ingredients:

- 5 carrots, sliced
- 1 and ½ cups great northern beans, dried, soaked overnight and drained
- 2 garlic cloves, minced
- 1 yellow onion, chopped
- Salt and black pepper to the taste
- ½ teaspoon oregano, dried
- 5 ounces baby spinach
- 4 and ½ cups veggie stock
- 2 teaspoons lemon peel, grated
- 3 tablespoons lemon juice
- 1 avocado, pitted, peeled and chopped
- ¾ cup tofu, firm, pressed, drained and crumbled
- ¼ cup pistachios, chopped

Directions:

1. In your slow cooker, mix beans with onion, carrots, garlic, salt, pepper, oregano and veggie stock, stir, cover and cook on High for 4 hours.
2. Drain beans mix, return to your slow cooker and reserve ¼ cup cooking liquid.
3. Add spinach, lemon juice and lemon peel, stir and leave aside for 5 minutes.
4. Transfer beans, carrots and spinach mixture to a bowl, add pistachios, avocado, tofu and reserve cooking liquid, toss, divide between plates and serve as a side dish.
5. Enjoy!

Scalloped Potatoes

Preparation time: 10 minutes

Cooking time: 4 hours

Servings: 8

Nutritional Values (Per Serving):

- Calories 306
- Fat 14
- Fiber 4
- Carbs 30
- Protein 12

Ingredients:

- Cooking spray
- 2 pounds gold potatoes, halved and sliced
- 1 yellow onion, cut into medium wedges
- 10 ounces canned vegan potato cream soup
- 8 ounces coconut milk

- 1 cup tofu, crumbled
- ½ cup veggie stock
- Salt and black pepper to the taste
- 1 tablespoons parsley, chopped

Directions:

1. Coat your slow cooker with cooking spray and arrange half of the potatoes on the bottom.
2. Layer onion wedges, half of the vegan cream soup, coconut milk, tofu, stock, salt and pepper.
3. Add the rest of the potatoes, onion wedges, cream, coconut milk, tofu and stock, cover and cook on High for 4 hours.
4. Sprinkle parsley on top, divide scalloped potatoes between plates and serve as a side dish.
5. Enjoy!

Sweet Potatoes Side Dish

Preparation time: 10 minutes

Cooking time: 3 hours

Servings: 10

Nutritional Values (Per Serving):

- Calories 189
- Fat 4
- Fiber 4
- Carbs 36
- Protein 4

Ingredients:

- 4 pounds sweet potatoes, thinly sliced
- 3 tablespoons stevia
- ½ cup orange juice
- A pinch of salt and black pepper
- ½ teaspoon thyme, dried

- ½ teaspoon sage, dried
- 2 tablespoons olive oil

Directions:

1. Arrange potato slices on the bottom of your slow cooker.
2. In a bowl, mix orange juice with salt, pepper, stevia, thyme, sage and oil and whisk well.
3. Add this over potatoes, cover slow cooker and cook on High for 3 hours.
4. Divide between plates and serve as a side dish.
5. Enjoy!

Cauliflower and Broccoli Side Dish

Preparation time: 10 minutes

Cooking time: 3 hours

Servings: 10

Nutritional Values (Per Serving):

- Calories 177
- Fat 12
- Fiber 2
- Carbs 10
- Protein 7

Ingredients:

- 4 cups broccoli florets
- 4 cups cauliflower florets
- 14 ounces tomato paste

- 1 yellow onion, chopped
- 1 teaspoon thyme, dried
- Salt and black pepper to the taste
- ½ cup almonds, sliced

Directions:

1. In your slow cooker, mix broccoli with cauliflower, tomato paste, onion, thyme, salt and pepper, toss, cover and cook on High for 3 hours.
2. Add almonds, toss, divide between plates and serve as a side dish.
3. Enjoy!

Wild Rice Mix

Preparation time: 10 minutes

Cooking time: 6 hours

Servings: 12

Nutritional Values (Per Serving):

- Calories 169
- Fat 5
- Fiber 3
- Carbs 28
- Protein 5

Ingredients:

- 40 ounces veggie stock
- 2 and ½ cups wild rice
- 1 cup carrot, shredded
- 4 ounces mushrooms, sliced
- 2 tablespoons olive oil

- 2 teaspoons marjoram, dried and crushed
- Salt and black pepper to the taste
- 2/3 cup dried cherries
- ½ cup pecans, toasted and chopped
- 2/3 cup green onions, chopped

Directions:

1. In your slow cooker, mix stock with wild rice, carrot, mushrooms, oil, marjoram, salt, pepper, cherries, pecans and green onions, toss, cover and cook on Low for 6 hours.
2. Stir wild rice one more time, divide between plates and serve as a side dish.
3. Enjoy!

Rustic Mashed Potatoes

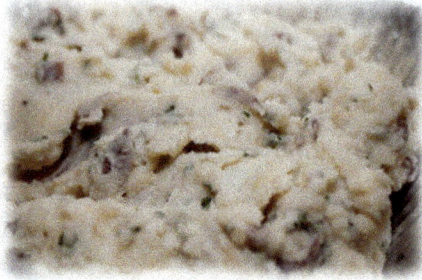

Preparation time: 10 minutes

Cooking time: 4 hours

Servings: 6

Nutritional Values (Per Serving):

- Calories 135
- Fat 5
- Fiber 1
- Carbs 20
- Protein 3

Ingredients:

- 6 garlic cloves, peeled
- 3 pounds gold potatoes, peeled and cubed
- 1 bay leaf
- 1 cup coconut milk
- 28 ounces veggie stock
- 3 tablespoons olive oil
- Salt and black pepper to the taste

Directions:

1. In your slow cooker, mix potatoes with stock, bay leaf, garlic, salt and pepper, cover and cook on High for 4 hours.
2. Drain potatoes and garlic, return them to your slow cooker and mash using a potato masher.
3. Add oil and coconut milk, whisk well, divide between plates and serve as a side dish.
4. Enjoy!

Fresh Fruit Smoothie

Preparation time: 5 mins

Servings: 4

Nutritional Values (Per Serving)

Calories: 72

Fat:1 g

Carbs:17 g

Protein:1 g

Sugars:1 g

Sodium:42 mg

Ingredients:

- 1 tbsp. honey
- ½ c. cantaloupe
- 1 c. water
- 1 c. fresh strawberries
- 1 c. fresh pineapple
- 2 orange juice

Directions:

1. Remove the rind from the melon and pineapple. Cut them into chunks and remove the stems from the strawberries.
2. Put everything in a blender and serve.

Popovers

Preparation time: 5 mins

Servings: 6

Nutritional Values (Per Serving):

- Calories: 101
- Fat:0 g
- Carbs:18 g
- Protein:6 g
- Sugars:2 g
- Sodium:125 mg

Ingredients:

- 4 egg whites
- 1 c. All-purpose flour
- 1 c. fat-free milk
- ¼ tsp. salt

Directions:

1. Preheat your oven to 425 0F.

2. Coat a six cup metal or glass muffin mold with cooking spray and heat the mold in the oven for two minutes.

3. In a bowl, add the flour, milk, salt, and egg whites. Use a mixer to beat until it's smooth.

4. Fill the heated molds two-thirds of the way full.

5. Bake until the muffins are golden brown and puffy, around half an hour. Serve.

Broccoli, Garlic, and Rigatoni

Preparation time: 10 mins

Servings: 2

Nutritional Values (Per Serving):

- Calories: 355
- Fat:7 g
- Carbs:63 g
- Protein:14 g
- Sugars:4 g
- Sodium:600 mg

Ingredients:

- 2 tsps. Minced garlic 2 c. Broccoli florets
- Freshly ground black pepper
- 2 tbsps. Parmesan cheese
- 1/3 lb. Rigatoni noodles
- 2 tsps. Olive oil

Directions:

1. Fill a pot three-quarters of the way full with water and bring it to a boil. Add the rigatoni and cook until it is firm, around twelve minutes. Drain it thoroughly.
2. As the pasta cooks, bring an inch of water to a boil and put a steamer basket over the top. Add the broccoli and steam for ten minutes.
3. In a bowl, mix together the pasta and broccoli. Toss with the cheese, oil, and garlic.
4. Season to taste and serve.

Vegan Rice Pudding

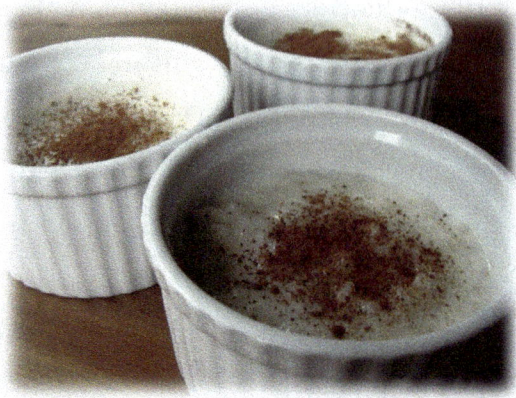

Preparation time: 5 mins

Servings: 8

Nutritional Values (Per Serving):

- Calories: 148
- Fat:2 g
- Carbs:26 g
- Protein:4 g
- Sugars:35 g
- Sodium:150 mg

Ingredients:

- ½ tsp. ground cinnamon
- 1 c. rinsed basmati
- 1/8 tsp. ground cardamom
- ¼ c. sugar
- 1/8 tsp. pure almond extract
- 1 quart vanilla nondairy milk
- 1 tsp. pure vanilla extract

Directions:

1. Measure all of the ingredients into a saucepan and stir well to combine. Bring to a boil over medium- high heat.
2. Once boiling, reduce heat to low and simmer, stirring very frequently, about 15–20 minutes.
3. Remove from heat and cool. Serve sprinkled with additional ground cinnamon if desired.

Cinnamon-Scented Quinoa

Preparation time: 5 mins

Servings: 4

Nutritional Values (Per Serving)

- Calories: 160
- Fat:3 g
- Carbs:28 g
- Protein:6 g
- Sugars:19 g
- Sodium:40 mg

Ingredients:

- Chopped walnuts
- 1 ½ c. water
- Maple syrup
- 2 cinnamon sticks
- 1 c. quinoa

Directions:

1. Add the quinoa to a bowl and wash it in several changes of water until the water is clear. When washing quinoa, rub grains and allow them to settle before you pour off the water.
2. Use a large fine-mesh sieve to drain the quinoa. Prepare your pressure cooker with a trivet and steaming basket. Place the quinoa and the cinnamon sticks in the basket and pour the water.
3. Close and lock the lid. Cook at high pressure for 6 minutes. When the cooking time is up, release the pressure using the quick release method.
4. Fluff the quinoa with a fork and remove the cinnamon sticks. Divide the cooked quinoa among serving bowls and top with maple syrup and chopped walnuts.

Pumpkin-Pear Soup

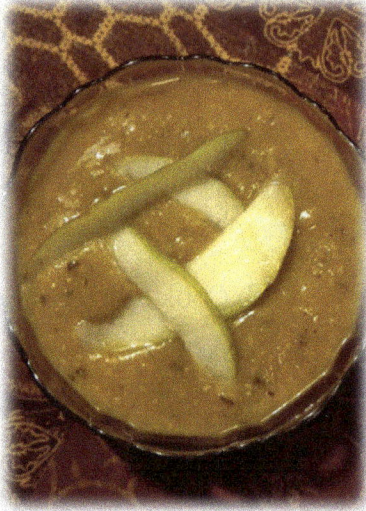

Preparation time: 10 Minutes

Cooking time: 15 Minutes

Servings: 4

Nutrition per Serving (2 cups)

- Calories: 90

- Protein: 2g
- Total fat: 1g
- Saturated fat: 0g
- Carbohydrates: 17g
- Fiber: 3g

Ingredients:

- 1 teaspoon olive oil or coconut oil
- 1 onion, diced, or 2 teaspoons onion powder
- 1-inch piece fresh ginger, peeled and diced, or 1 teaspoon ground ginger 1 pear, cored and chopped
- Optional spices to take the taste up a notch: 1 teaspoon curry powder
- ½ teaspoon pumpkin pie spice
- ½ teaspoon smoked paprika
- Pinch red pepper flakes
- 4 cups water or Economical Vegetable Broth
- 3 cups canned pumpkin purée
- 1 to 2 teaspoons salt (less if using salted broth)
- Pinch freshly ground black pepper
- ¼ to ½ cup canned coconut milk (optional)
- 2to 4 tablespoons nutritional yeast (optional)

Directions:

1. Preparing the ingredients

2. Heat the olive oil in a large pot over medium heat. Add the onion, ginger, and pear and sauté for about 5 minutes, until soft. Sprinkle in any optional spices and stir to combine.

3. Add the water, pumpkin, salt, and pepper, and stir until smooth and combined. Cook until just bubbling, about 10 minutes.

4. Stir in the coconut milk (if using) and nutritional yeast (if using), and remove the soup from the heat. Leftovers will keep in an airtight container for up to 1 week in the refrigerator or up to 1 month in the freezer.

Sweet Potato and Peanut Soup with Baby Spinach

Preparation time: 5 Minutes

Cooking time: 40 Minutes

Servings: 4

Ingredients:

- 1 tablespoon olive oil
- 1 medium onion, chopped
- 1½ pounds sweet potatoes, peeled and cut into ½-inch dice
- 6 cups vegetable broth (homemade, store-bought, or water)
- ⅓ cup creamy peanut butter
- ¼ teaspoon ground cayenne
- ⅛ teaspoon ground nutmeg
- Salt and freshly ground black pepper

- 4 cups fresh baby spinach

Directions:

1. In a large soup pot, heat the oil over medium heat. Add the onion, cover, and cook until softened, about 5 minutes. Add the sweet potatoes and broth and cook, uncovered, until the potatoes are tender, about 30 minutes.
2. Ladle about a cup of hot broth into a small bowl. Add the peanut butter and stir until smooth. Stir the peanut butter mixture into the soup along with the cayenne, nutmeg, and salt and pepper to taste.
3. About 10 minutes before ready to serve, stir in the spinach, and serve.

Tuscan White Bean Soup

Preparation time: 10 Minutes

Cooking time: 15 Minutes

Servings: 4

- Nutrition per Serving (2 cups)
- Calories: 145
- Protein: 7g
- Total fat: 2g
- Saturated fat: 0g
- Carbohydrates: 26g
- Fiber: 6g

Ingredients:

- 1 to 2 teaspoons olive oil
- 1 onion, chopped
- 4 garlic cloves, minced, or 1 teaspoon garlic powder
- 2 carrots, peeled and chopped
- Salt
- 1 tablespoon dried herbs

- Pinch freshly ground black pepper
- Pinch red pepper flakes
- 4 cups Economical Vegetable Broth or water
- 2 (15-ounce) cans white beans, such as cannellini, navy, or great northern, drained and rinsed
- 2 tablespoons freshly squeezed lemon juice
- 2 cups chopped greens, such as spinach, kale, arugula, or chard

Directions:

1. Preparing the ingredients
2. Heat the olive oil in a large soup pot over medium-high heat.
3. Add the onion, garlic (if using fresh), carrots, and a pinch of salt.
4. Sauté for about 5 minutes, stirring occasionally, until the vegetables are lightly browned. Sprinkle in the dried herbs (plus the garlic powder, if using), black pepper, and red pepper flakes, and toss to combine.
5. Add the vegetable broth, beans, and another pinch of salt, and bring the soup to a low simmer to heat through. If you like, make the broth a bit creamier by puréeing 1 to 2 cups of soup in a countertop blender and returning it to

the pot. Alternatively, use a hand blender to purée about one-fourth of the beans in the pot.

6. Stir in the lemon juice and greens, and let the greens wilt into the soup before serving. Leftovers will keep in an airtight container for up to 1 week in the refrigerator or up to 1 month in the freezer.

Thai Tofu Shirataki Stir-Fry

Preparation time: 35 minutes

Serving: 4

Nutritional Values (Per Serving):

- Calories: 598
- Total Fat: 56g
- Saturated Fat:18.8g
- Total Carbs: 12 g
- Dietary Fiber3:g
- Sugar:5 g
- Protein: 15g
- Sodium:762 mg

Ingredients:

For the angel hair shirataki:

- 2 (8 oz) packs angel hair shirataki

For the teriyaki tofu base:

- 2 tbsp olive oil, divided
- 1 ¼ lb tofu, cut into bite-size pieces
- Salt and black pepper to taste
- 1 white onion, thinly sliced
- 1 red bell pepper, deseeded and sliced
- 1 cup sliced cremini mushrooms
- 4 garlic cloves, minced
- 1 ½ cups fresh Thai basil leaves
- 2 tbsp toasted sesame seeds
- 1 tbsp chopped peanuts
- 1 tbsp chopped fresh scallions

For the sauce:

- 3 tbsp coconut aminos
- 2 tbsp Himalayan salt
- 1 tbsp hot sauce

Directions:

For the angel hair shirataki:

1. Boil 2 cups of water in a medium pot over medium heat.
2. Strain the shirataki pasta through a colander and rinse very well under hot running water.
3. Allow proper draining and pour the shirataki pasta into the boiling water. Cook for 3 minutes and strain again.
4. Place a dry skillet over medium heat and stir-fry the shirataki pasta until visibly dry, and makes a squeaky sound when stirred, 1 to 2 minutes. Take off the heat and set aside.

For the teriyaki tofu base:

5. Heat the olive oil in a large skillet, season the tofu with salt, black pepper, and sear in the oil on both sides until brown, 5 minutes. Transfer to a plate and set aside.
6. Add the onion, bell pepper, and mushrooms to the skillet; cook until softened, 5 minutes. Stir in the garlic and cook until fragrant, 1 minute.
7. Return the tofu to the skillet and add the pasta.
8. Quickly, combine the sauce's ingredients in a small bowl: coconut aminos, Himalayan salt, and hot sauce. Pour the mixture over the tofu mix. Top with the Thai basil and

toss well to coat. Cook for 1 to 2 minutes or until warmed through.

9. Dish the food onto serving plates and garnish with the sesame seeds, peanuts, and scallions.

Classic Tempeh Lasagna

Preparation time: 70 minutes

Serving: 4

Nutritional Values (Per Serving):

- Calories:43
- Total Fat:38.3g
- Saturated Fat:1.2g
- Total Carbs: 4 g
- Dietary Fiber:1g
- Sugar: 2g,
- Protein21: g
- Sodium: 388mg

Ingredients:

For the lasagna noodles:

- 4 oz dairy- free cream cheese, room temperature
- 1 ½ cup grated mozzarella cheese

- 1 tsp dried Italian seasoning
- 2 large eggs, cracked into a bowl

For the lasagna filling:

- 1 lb tempeh
- 1 medium white onion, chopped
- 1 tsp Italian seasoning
- Salt and black pepper to taste
- 1 cup sugar-free marinara sauce
- 6 tbsp vegan ricotta cheese
- ½ cup grated mozzarella cheese
- ½ cup grated parmesan cheese

Directions:

For the lasagna noodles:

1. Preheat the oven to 350 F and line a 9 x 13 –inch baking sheet with parchment paper.
2. In a food processor or blender, add the dairy- free cream cheese, mozzarella cheese, Italian seasoning, and eggs. Blend until well mixed.
3. Pour the cheese mixture on the baking sheet and spread across the pan.

4. Bake in the middle layer of the oven until set and firm to touch, 20 minutes.

5. Remove the cheese pasta and set aside to cool while you make the lasagna sauce.

For the lasagna sauce:

6. In a large skillet, combine the tempeh, onion and cook until brown, 5 minutes. Season with the Italian seasoning, salt, and black pepper. Cook further for 1 minute and mix in the marinara sauce. Simmer for 3 minutes. Turn the heat off.

7. Evenly cut the lasagna pasta into thirds making sure it fits into your baking sheet.

8. Spread a layer of the tempeh mixture in the baking sheet and make a first single layer on the tempeh mixture.

9. Spread a third of the remaining tempeh mixture on the pasta, top with a third each of the vegan ricotta cheese, mozzarella cheese, and parmesan cheese. Repeat the layering two more times using the remaining ingredients in the same quantities.

10. Bake in the oven until the cheese melts and is bubbly with the sauce, 20 minutes. Serve warm.

11. Remove the lasagna, allow cooling for 2 minutes and dish onto serving plates.

Yellow Mung Bean Salad with Broccoli and Mango

Preparation time: 5 Minutes

Cooking time: 20 Minutes

Servings: 4

Ingredients:

- 1/2 cup yellow mung beans, picked over, rinsed, and drained
- 3 cups small broccoli florets, blanched
- 1 ripe mango, peeled, pitted, and chopped
- 1 small red bell pepper, chopped
- 1 jalapeño or other hot green chile, seeded and minced
- 2 tablespoons chopped fresh cilantro
- 1 teaspoon grated fresh ginger
- 2 tablespoons fresh lemon juice
- 3 tablespoons grapeseed oil

- 1/3 cup unsalted roasted cashews, for garnish

Directions:

1. In a saucepan of boiling salted water, cook the mung beans until just tender, 18 to 20 minutes. Drain and run under cold water to cool. Transfer the beans to a large bowl. Add the broccoli, mango, bell pepper, chile, and cilantro. Set aside.
2. In a small bowl, combine the ginger, lemon juice, oil. Stir to mix well, then pour the dressing over the vegetables and toss to combine. Sprinkle with cashews and serve.

Asian Slaw

Preparation time: 15 Minutes

Cooking time: 0 Minutes

Servings: 4

Ingredients:

- 8 ounces napa cabbage, cut crosswise into 1/4-inch strips
- 1 cup grated carrot
- 1 cup grated daikon radish
- 2 green onions, minced
- 2 tablespoons chopped fresh parsley
- 2 tablespoons rice vinegar
- 1 tablespoon grapeseed oil
- 2 teaspoons toasted sesame oil
- 1 tablespoon soy sauce
- 1 teaspoon grated fresh ginger
- 1/2 teaspoon dry mustard
- Salt and freshly ground black pepper

- 2 tablespoons chopped unsalted roasted peanuts, for garnish (optional)

Directions:

1. In a large bowl, combine the napa cabbage, carrot, daikon, green onions, and parsley. Set aside.
2. In a small bowl, combine the vinegar, grapeseed oil, sesame oil, soy sauce, ginger, mustard, and salt and pepper to taste. Stir until well blended. Pour the dressing over the vegetables and toss gently to coat. Taste, adjusting seasonings if necessary. Cover and refrigerate to allow flavors to blend, about 2 hours. Sprinkle with peanuts, if using, and serve.

The Great Green Salad

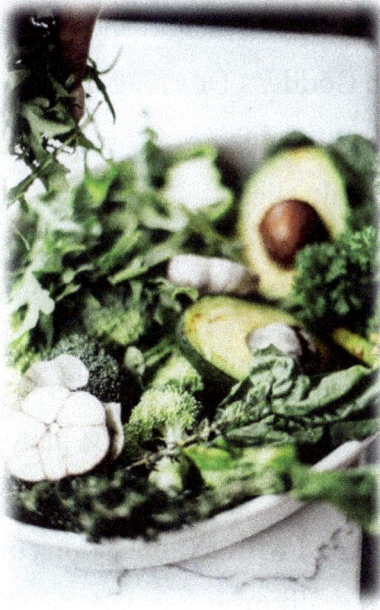

Preparation time: 10 Minutes

Cooking time: 0 Minutes

Servings: 4

Ingredients:

- 1 head Boston or Bibb lettuce
- 8 asparagus spears, trimmed and cut into 2-inch pieces

- 2 mini seedless cucumbers, sliced
- 1 small zucchini, cut into ribbons with potato peeler
- 1 avocado, peeled, pitted, and sliced
- ½ cup Green Goddess Dressing or store-bought vegan green goddess dressing
- 2 scallions, thinly sliced

Directions:

1. Divide the lettuce leaves among 4 plates. Top each with some of the asparagus, cucumber, zucchini, and avocado. Drizzle each bowl with 2 tablespoons of dressing and sprinkle with scallions.

Baked Hot Spicy Cashews Snack

Preparation time: 20 minutes

Cooking time: 35 minutes

Servings: 8

Nutritional Values (Per Serving):

- Calories: 41
- Fat: 29.01g
- Carbs: 9.6g
- Protein: 6.71g

Ingredients:

- 2½ c. raw cashews
- 1/3 c. olive oil
- ½ tsp. turmeric powder
- 1 tsp. garlic powder

- 3 c. hot pepper sauce

Directions:

1. In a mixing bowl, mix hot pepper sauce, oil and stir in the turmeric and garlic powder.
2. Add the cashews to the bowl and completely coat with hot pepper sauce mixture.
3. Soak cashews in the hot sauce mixture for several hours.
4. Preheat oven to 325F.
5. Spread the cashews onto a baking sheet and bake for 35-35 minutes.
6. Allow cool and serve.

Easy Avocado and Cremini Mushroom Melts

Preparation time: 15 minutes

Cooking time: 25 minutes

Servings: 4

Nutritional Values (Per Serving):

- Calories: 77
- Fat: 16.25g
- Carbs: 11.35g
- Protein: 9.32g

Ingredients:

- 8 sliced Cremini mushrooms
- 1 tbsp. olive oil
- 1 c. guacamole
- 1 tbsp. balsamic vinegar

- 12 slices cheddar cheese
- 3 slices Keto bread
- Salt Pepper

Directions:

1. Preheat oven to 350°F.
2. Using a skillet, Sauté balsamic vinegar, mushrooms, and olive oil medium high heat for 15 minutes, as you stir oftenly, until mushrooms are fragrant and golden brown.
3. Spread guacamole on bread and top with sautéed cheese and mushrooms.
4. Bake for approximately 10 minutes and ensure all the cheese melts out.
5. Serve and enjoy!

Keto Hot Peppers C.s

Preparation time: 15 minutes

Cooking time: 15-20 minutes

Servings: 4

Nutritional Values (Per Serving):

- Calories: 35
- Fat: 11.65g
- Carbs: 16.33g
- Protein: 12.57g

Ingredients:

- 4 eggs, beaten
- 3 hot red peppers, dried
- 8 tbsps. buckwheat flour
- 2 tsps. baking powder
- 2½ tbsps. coconut milk
- 4 freshly chopped basil leaves

- 1 tbsp. olive oil
- ½ tsp. salt

Directions:

1. Preheat oven to 380F.
2. In a bowl, mix the eggs, coconut milk, fresh basil and hot peppers.
3. In a separate mixing bowl, mix the buckwheat flour with the baking powder and salt.
4. Unite the egg mixture with the flour mixture and stir well.
5. Pour the batter in cups (3/4 c. full).
6. Bake in oven for 15-20 minutes.
7. When ready let cool and serve.

Spanish Vegetable Omelet

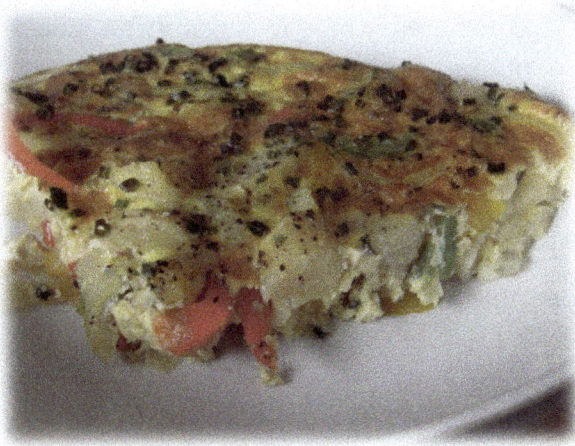

Preparation time: 10 minutes

Cooking time: 15 minutes

Servings: 4

Nutritional Values (Per Serving):

- Calories: 0
- Fat: 7.53g
- Carbs: 6.7
- Protein: 10.91g

Ingredients:

- 6 eggs
- 2 red peppers, chopped in thin strips
- 3 tbsps. olive oil
- 2 chopped scallions
- 1 diced zucchini Salt
- Black pepper

Directions:

1. Heat the olive oil in a pan; sauté chopped green onions for 3-4 minutes.
2. Add the peppers and cook for about 2 minutes more.
3. Add the zucchini and sauté for another 3 minutes.
4. In a mixing bowl, beat the eggs. Add salt and pepper to taste.
5. Mix the vegetables into the eggs.
6. Heat the olive oil in the frying pan and pour the whisked eggs mixture into the skillet.
7. Cook the omelet for 1 to 2 minutes. Serve hot.

Absolute Avocado Pizza

Preparation time: 10 minutes

Cooking time: 25 minutes

Servings: 4

Nutritional Values (Per Serving):

- Calories: 65
- Fat: 20.87g
- Carbs: 1.22g
- Protein: 18.27g

Ingredients:

Dough

- 2 eggs
- 4 tbsps. grated Parmesan cheese
- 2 envelopes unflavored gelatin
- ½ c. unsweetened Greek yogurt
- 4 tbsps. water

- 3 tbsps. grass-fed butter
- Salt

Filling

- Cheese, mushrooms, avocado puree, chopped fresh parsley

Directions:

1. Preheat oven to 450 degrees F.
2. Place all ingredients in a blender (gelatin without dissolving and beat well.
3. Grease a parchment paper with butter and evenly distribute the dough.
4. Place dough in greased baking pan and bake about 15 minutes.
5. Remove pizza from the oven and spread evenly with avocado sauce.
6. Top with your favorite fillings and sprinkle with the cheese.
7. Bake for 5 -10 minutes.
8. Remove from oven, let rest for 5 minutes and slice.
9. Serve immediately.

Almond Lemon Biscuits

Preparation time: 10 minutes

Cooking time: 12-15 minutes

Servings: 6

Nutritional Values (Per Serving):

- Calories: 27
- Fat: 25.91g
- Carbs: 4.49g
- Protein 5.9g

Ingredients:

- 3 c. almond flour
- ½ c. unsalted grass-fed butter
- 2 eggs
- 1 tbsp. fresh lemon juice
- 3 tbsps. Stevia
- 1½ tsps. Baking powder

Directions:

1. Preheat oven to 350F.
2. Combine the almond flour, Stevia and baking powder in a bowl.
3. Whisk the eggs in a separate bowl.
4. Melt the butter, and combine with almond flour, lemon juice and eggs mixture; stir well.
5. Divide mixture equally into 6 biscuits and place in a greased baking dish.
6. Bake for 12-15 minutes.
7. Let cool on a wire rack.
8. Serve warm or cold.

DESSERTS

Low-Carb Curd Soufflé

Preparation time: 45 minutes

Ingredients:

For the soufflé:

- 7 Oz. cream
- ½ cup condensed milk
- 1 pack (1 Oz.) gelatin for a dense soufflé
- 1 cup milk
- 5 Oz. cottage cheese

Directions:

1. Fill the gelatin with milk and set aside.
2. Mix the condensed milk with the cream and bring to boil on a low heat.
3. Pour the gelatin mass into the boiled mixture and mix it, then let it cool.

4. In a mixer, have all the mass combined well with the cottage cheese for at least 10 minutes.
1. Pour it into the silicone moulds for the cupcakes and let it freeze for a couple of hours and serve.

Cream Cheese Cookies

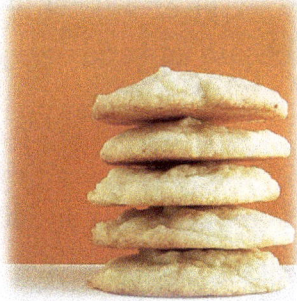

Preparation time: 40 minutes

Ingredients:

- 1 cup butter
- ¾ cup stevia or any sugar substitute
- 4 Oz. cream cheese, softened
- 1 egg
- 2 cups almond flour
- 1 cup coconut flour
- Sesame seeds
- Vanilla or any flavored extract to taste

Directions:

1. Mix the butter with the sweetener until fluffy.
2. Beat the cream cheese and add the egg, then flour and mix it with the flavor and seeds you have chosen.
3. Let it chill for 3-4 hours.
4. Roll the cookie mass into a log and have it sliced thus forming your cookies.
5. Bake until brown up to 15 minutes or more to make them crispy.

Chia Seeds Pudding with Berries

Preparation time: 60 minutes

Ingredients:

- 2 cups coconut milk, full fat
- 1 banana, sliced
- ½ cups chia seeds
- Honey or stevia for sweetening
- 5 Oz. at least any fresh berries

Directions:

1. Stir the milk, chia seeds and stevia (or honey) in a mixing bowl.
2. Add half of all the berries and let the mixture chilled for at least 1 hour.
3. Mix it up again and add the berries and banana before serving.

Tip: Chia seeds have omega-3 fatty acids, protein, fiber, calcium and antioxidants.

Smoothie Bowl

Preparation time: 45 minutes

Ingredients:

- 6 Oz. berries, fresh or frozen
- 2 medium frozen bananas
- ½ cup Almond milk
- 1 cup jellified yoghurt
- 1 tbsp. Chia seeds
- 1 tbsp. Hemp seeds
- 1 tbsp. Coconut flakes
- Raspberry jam or any other, to taste

Directions:

1. In a blender mix the bananas with half of the berries until it has a puree consistency.
2. Organise your smoothie in a bowl decorating it in rows with the yogurt spot, the puree and fresh berries and with a pinch of seeds and flakes you have.

Coconut milk smoothie

Preparation time: 15 minutes

Ingredients:

- 1 cup Greek yogurt
- 1 cup coconut milk, full fat
- 1 banana, fresh or frozen
- 1 cup baby spinach, fresh
- 1 tbsp. honey
- 5 Oz. blueberries or other berries

Directions:

1. In a blender mix all the ingredients until smooth. Add the ice for a thicker smoothie.

Yogurt Smoothie with Cinnamon and Mango

Preparation time: 15 minutes

Ingredients:

- 4 Oz. frozen mango chunks, mango pulp or fresh mango 1 cup Greek yogurt
- 1 cup coconut milk, full fat
- 3-4 cups milk
- 3 tbsp. flax seed meal
- 1 tbsp. honey
- 1 tsp. cinnamon

Directions:

1. In a blender mix all the ingredients, except cinnamon until smooth. Sprinkle each smoothie with a pinch of cinnamon.

Lemon Curd Dessert (Sugar Free)

Preparation time: 35 minutes

Ingredients:

- ½ cup unsalted butter
- ½ cup lemon juice
- 2 tbsp. lemon zest
- 6 egg yolks
- Stevia for sweetening

Directions:

1. On a low heat melt the butter in a saucepan.
2. Whisk in the stevia or any other sweetener, lemon ingredients until combined, then add the egg yolks and return to the stove again over the low heat.
3. Whisk it until the curd starts thickening.
4. Strain into a small bowl and let cool.
5. Can be stored in a fridge for several weeks.

Chocolate Almond Butter Smoothie

Preparation time: 35 minutes

Ingredients:

- 2 tbsp. chocolate protein powder
- ½ tbsp. cacao powder
- 1 cup almond milk
- 2 tbsp. almond butter
- 1 fresh banana
- ½ cup fresh strawberries
- 1 tbsp. chia or hemp seeds
- Maple syrup or stevia for sweetening

Directions:

1. Put all the ingredients into the blender and mix until it has creamy consistency.

Vegan Gumbo

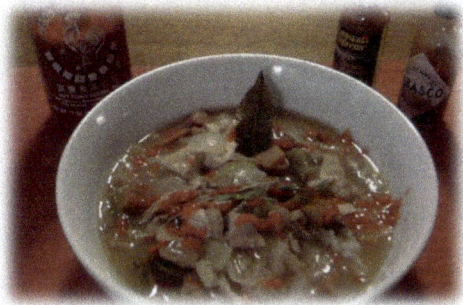

Preparation time: 10 minutes

Cooking time: 8 hours

Servings: 4

Nutritions:

- Calories 312
- Fat 4
- Fiber 7
- Carbs 19
- Protein 4

Ingredients:

- 2 tablespoons olive oil
- 1 green bell pepper, chopped
- 1 yellow onion, chopped
- 2 celery stalks, chopped
- 3 garlic cloves, minced
- 15 ounces canned tomatoes, chopped
- 2 cups veggie stock
- 8 ounces white mushrooms, sliced
- 15 ounces canned kidney beans, drained
- 1 zucchini, chopped
- 1 tablespoon Cajun seasoning
- Salt and black pepper to the taste

Directions:

1. In your slow cooker, mix oil with bell pepper, onion, celery, garlic, tomatoes, stock, mushrooms, beans, zucchini, Cajun seasoning, salt and pepper, stir, cover and cook on Low for 8 hours
2. Divide into bowls and serve hot.
3. Enjoy!

Eggplant Salad

Preparation time: 10 minutes

Cooking time: 8 hours

Servings: 4

Nutritions:

- Calories 251
- Fat 4
- Fiber 6
- Carbs 8
- Protein 3

Ingredients:

- 24 ounces canned tomatoes, chopped
- 1 red onion, chopped
- 2 red bell peppers, chopped
- 1 big eggplant, roughly chopped
- 1 tablespoon smoked paprika

- 2 teaspoons cumin, ground
- Salt and black pepper to the taste
- Juice of 1 lemon
- 1 tablespoons parsley, chopped

Directions:

1. In your slow cooker, mix tomatoes with onion, bell peppers, eggplant, smoked paprika, cumin, salt, pepper and lemon juice, stir, cover and cook on Low for 8 hours
2. Add parsley, stir, divide into bowls and serve cold as a dinner salad.
3. Enjoy!

Corn and Cabbage Soup

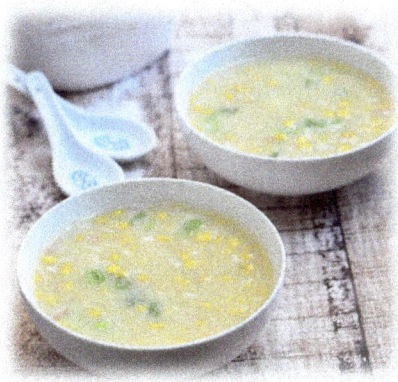

Preparation time: 10 minutes

Cooking time: 7 hours

Servings: 4

Nutritions:

- Calories 300
- Fat 4
- Fiber 4
- Carbs 10
- Protein 4

Ingredients:

- 1 small yellow onion, chopped
- 1 tablespoon olive oil
- 2 garlic cloves, minced
- 1 and ½ cups mushrooms, sliced
- 3 teaspoons ginger, grated
- A pinch of salt and black pepper
- 2 cups corn kernels
- 4 cups red cabbage, chopped
- 4 cups water
- 1 tablespoon nutritional yeast
- 2 teaspoons tomato paste
- 1 teaspoon sesame oil
- 1 teaspoon coconut aminos
- 1 teaspoon sriracha sauce

Directions:

1. In your slow cooker, mix olive oil with onion, garlic, mushrooms, ginger, salt, pepper, corn, cabbage, water,

yeast and tomato paste, stir, cover and cook on Low for 7 hours.

2. Add sriracha sauce and aminos, stir, leave soup aside for a few minutes, ladle into bowls, drizzle sesame oil all over and serve.

3. Enjoy!

Okra Soup

Preparation time: 10 minutes

Cooking time: 5 hours

Servings: 6

Nutritions:

- Calories 243
- Fat 4
- Fiber 6
- Carbs 10
- Protein 3

Ingredients:

- 1 green bell pepper, chopped
- 1 small yellow onion, chopped
- 3 cups veggie stock
- 3 garlic cloves, minced
- 16 ounces okra, sliced

- 2 cup corn
- 29 ounces canned tomatoes, crushed
- 1 and ½ teaspoon smoked paprika
- 1 teaspoon marjoram, dried
- 1 teaspoon thyme, dried
- 1 teaspoon oregano, dried
- Salt and black pepper to the taste

Directions:

1. In your slow cooker, mix bell pepper with onion, stock, garlic, okra, corn, tomatoes, smoked paprika, marjoram, thyme, oregano, salt and pepper, stir, cover and cook on High for 5 hours.
2. Ladle into bowls and serve.
3. Enjoy!

Carrot Soup

Preparation time: 10 minutes

Cooking time: 5 hours

Servings: 6

Nutritions:

- calories 241
- fat 4
- fiber 7
- carbs 10
- protein 4

Ingredients:

- 2 potatoes, cubed
- 3 pounds carrots, cubed
- 1 yellow onion, chopped
- 1-quart veggie stock
- Salt and black pepper to the taste

- 1 teaspoon thyme, dried
- 3 tablespoons coconut milk
- 2 teaspoons curry powder
- 3 tablespoons vegan cheese, crumbled
- A handful pistachios, chopped

Directions:

1. In your slow cooker, mix onion with potatoes, carrots, stock, salt, pepper, thyme and curry powder, stir, cover, cook on High for 1 hour and on Low for 4 hours.
2. Add coconut milk, stir, blend soup using an immersion blender, ladle soup into bowls, sprinkle vegan cheese and pistachios on top and serve.
3. Enjoy!

Baby Carrots and Coconut Soup

Preparation time: 10 minutes

Cooking time: 7 hours

Servings: 6

Nutritions:

- Calories 100
- Fat 2
- Fiber 4
- Carbs 18
- Protein 3

Ingredients:

- 1 sweet potato, cubed
- 2 pounds baby carrots, peeled
- 2 teaspoons ginger paste
- 1 yellow onion, chopped
- 4 cups veggie stock

- 2 teaspoons curry powder
- Salt and black pepper to the taste
- 14 ounces coconut milk

Directions:

1. In your slow cooker, mix sweet potato with baby carrots, ginger paste, onion, stock, curry powder, salt and pepper, stir, cover and cook on High for 7 hours.
2. Add coconut milk, blend soup using an immersion blender, divide soup into bowls and serve.
3. Enjoy!

www.ingramcontent.com/pod-product-compliance
Lightning Source LLC
Chambersburg PA
CBHW050751030426
42336CB00012B/1764

9 781802 772128